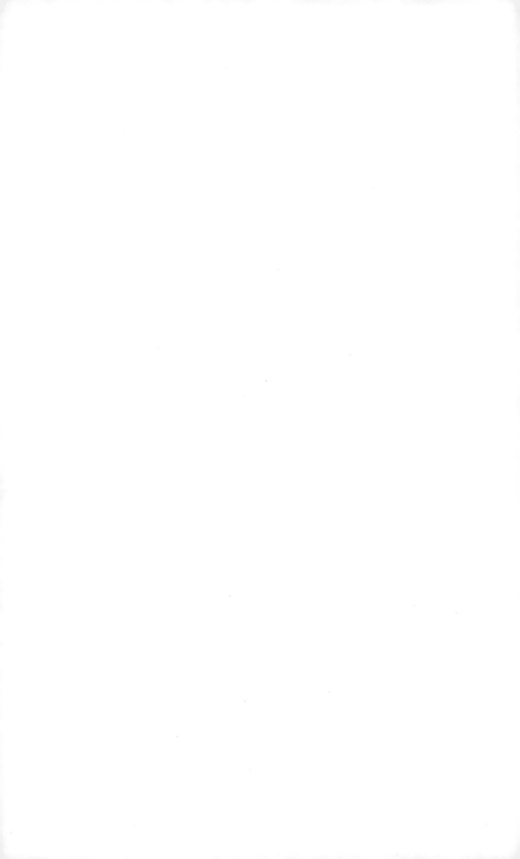

The Mediterranean Beginners' Cooking Guide

A Handful Of Quick, Delicious Recipes for
Your Mediterranean Meals

Dan Peterson

TABLE OF CONTENT

result of the use of information contained within this document, including, but not limited to, — errors, omissions, or inaccuracies.

Bacon-Wrapped Chicken

Preparation Time: 10 minutes

Cooking Time: 50 minutes

Servings: 2

INGREDIENTS:
- 4 slices Bacon
- Salt
- Pepper
- 4 oz. or 113 g. Cheddar Cheese, grated
- 2 Chicken Breasts
- Paprika to taste
- 2 tbsps. lemon or orange fresh juice

DIRECTIONS:
1. Heat the oven to 350 F/ 176 C.
2. Place chicken breasts into a medium bowl and season with salt, pepper, paprika, and fresh juice.
3. Replace chicken breasts to a baking pan.
4. Add cheese on top and place bacon slices over chicken breasts.
5. Place the baking pan to the oven for 45 minutes.
6. Take away from the oven your dish and the double-meat meal are ready to be served.
7. Note: If you want to get extra crispy bacon, place your cooked breasts covered with cheese and bacon on a grill or skillet and sauté for 2 minutes on each side.

NUTRITION: Calories 206, Fat 8 g, Sat. fat 3.7 g, Fiber 0 g, Carbs 1.6 g, Sugars 1.6 g, Protein 30 g, Sodium 302 mg

Broccoli Pesto Spaghetti

Preparation Time: 10 minutes
Cooking Time : 20 minutes

Servings: 2

INGREDIENTS:
- 8 oz. or 226.7g spaghetti
- 1 lb. or 450g broccoli, cut into florets
- 2 tbsps. olive oil
- 4 garlic cloves, chopped
- 4 basil leaves
- 2 tbsps. blanched almonds
- 1 juiced lemon
- Salt and pepper

DIRECTIONS:
1. For the pesto, combine the broccoli, oil, garlic, basil, lemon juice and almonds in a blender and pulse until well mixed and smooth.
2. Set spaghetti in a pot, add salt and pepper. Cook until al dente for about 8 minutes. Drain well.
3. Mix the warm spaghetti with the broccoli pesto and serve.

NUTRITION: Calories 284, Fat 10.2 g, Sat. fat 3 g, Fiber 10 g, Carbs 40.2 g, Sugar 6 g, Protein 10.4 g, Sodium 421 mg

Creamy Chicken Breasts

Preparation Time : 10 minutes
Cooking Time : 12 minutes

Servings: 4

INGREDIENTS:
- 4 chicken breasts, skinless and boneless
- 1 tbsp basil pesto
- 1 1/2 tbsp cornstarch
- 1/4 cup roasted red peppers, chopped
- 1/3 cup heavy cream
- 1 tsp Italian seasoning
- 1 tsp garlic, minced
- 1 cup chicken broth
- Pepper
- Salt

DIRECTIONS:
1. Add chicken into the instant pot. Season chicken with Italian seasoning, pepper, and salt. Sprinkle with garlic. Pour broth over chicken. Seal pot with lid and cook on high for 8 minutes.
2. Once done, allow to release pressure naturally for 5 minutes then release remaining using quick release. Remove lid. Transfer chicken on a plate and clean the instant pot.
3. Set instant pot on sauté mode. Add heavy cream, pesto, cornstarch, and red pepper to the pot and stir well and cook for 3-4 minutes.
4. Return chicken to the pot and coat well with the sauce. Serve and enjoy.

NUTRITION: Calories 341 Fat 15.2 g Carbohydrates 4.4 g Protein 43.8 g

Cheese Garlic Chicken & Potatoes

Preparation Time: 10 minutes

Cooking Time: 13 minutes

Servings: 4

INGREDIENTS:
- 2 lb. chicken breasts, skinless, boneless, cut into chunks
- 1 tbsp olive oil
- 3/4 cup chicken broth
- 1 tbsp Italian seasoning
- 1 tbsp garlic powder
- 1 tsp garlic, minced
- 1 1/2 cup parmesan cheese, shredded
- 1 lb. potatoes, chopped
- Pepper
- Salt

DIRECTIONS:
1. Add oil into the inner pot of instant pot and set the pot on sauté mode. Add chicken and cook until browned. Add remaining ingredients except for cheese and stir well.
2. Seal pot with lid and cook on high for 8 minutes. Once done, release pressure using quick release. Remove lid. Top with cheese and cover with lid for 5 minutes or until cheese is melted. Serve and enjoy.

NUTRITION: Calories 674 Fat 29 g Carbohydrates 21.4 g Protein 79.7 g

Easy Chicken Scampi

Preparation Time: 10 minutes

Cooking Time: 25 minutes

Servings: 4

INGREDIENTS:
- 3 chicken breasts, skinless, boneless, and sliced
- 1 tsp garlic, minced
- 1 tbsp Italian seasoning
- 2 cups chicken broth
- 1 bell pepper, sliced
- 1/2 onion, sliced
- Pepper
- Salt

DIRECTIONS:
1. Add chicken into the instant pot and top with remaining ingredients. Seal pot with lid and cook on high for 25 minutes. Once done, release pressure using quick release. Remove lid.
2. Remove chicken from pot and shred using a fork. Return shredded chicken to the pot and stir well. Serve over cooked whole grain pasta and top with cheese.

NUTRITION: Calories 254 Fat 9.9 g Carbohydrates 4.6 g Protein 34.6 g

Protein Packed Chicken Bean Rice

Preparation Time: 10 minutes

Cooking Time: 15 minutes

Servings: 6

INGREDIENTS:
- 1 lb. chicken breasts, skinless, boneless, and cut into chunks
- 14 oz can cannellini beans, rinsed and drained
- 4 cups chicken broth
- 2 cups brown rice
- 1 tbsp Italian seasoning
- 1 small onion, chopped
- 1 tbsp garlic, chopped
- 1 tbsp olive oil
- Pepper
- Salt

DIRECTIONS:
1. Add oil into the inner pot of instant pot and set the pot on sauté mode. Add garlic and onion and sauté for 3 minutes. Add remaining ingredients and stir everything well.
2. Seal pot with a lid and select manual and set timer for 12 minutes. Once done, release pressure using quick release. Remove lid. Stir well and serve.

NUTRITION: Calories 494 Fat 11.3 g Carbohydrates 61.4 g Protein 34.2 g

Pesto Vegetable Chicken

Preparation Time: 10 minutes

Cooking Time: 25 minutes

Servings: 4

INGREDIENTS:
- 1 1/2 lb. chicken thighs, skinless, boneless, and cut into pieces
- 1/2 cup chicken broth
- 1/4 cup fresh parsley, chopped
- 2 cups cherry tomatoes, halved
- 1 cup basil pesto
- 3/4 lb. asparagus, trimmed and cut in half
- 2/3 cup sun-dried tomatoes, drained and chopped
- 2 tbsp olive oil
- Pepper
- Salt

DIRECTIONS:
1. Add oil into the inner pot of instant pot and set the pot on sauté mode. Add chicken and sauté for 5 minutes. Add remaining ingredients except for tomatoes and stir well.
2. Seal pot with a lid and select manual and set timer for 15 minutes. Once done, release pressure using quick release. Remove lid.
3. Add tomatoes and stir well. Again, seal the pot and select manual and set timer for 5 minutes. Release pressure using quick release. Remove lid. Stir well and serve.

NUTRITION: Calories 459 Fat 20.5 g Carbohydrates 14.9 g Protein 9.2 g

Greek Chicken Rice

Preparation Time: 10 minutes

Cooking Time: 14 minutes

Servings: 4

INGREDIENTS:
- 3 chicken breasts, skinless, boneless, and cut into chunks
- 1/4 fresh parsley, chopped
- 1 zucchini, sliced
- 2 bell peppers, chopped
- 1 cup rice, rinsed and drained
- 1 1/2 cup chicken broth
- 1 tbsp oregano
- 3 tbsp fresh lemon juice
- 1 tbsp garlic, minced
- 1 onion, diced
- 2 tbsp olive oil
- Pepper
- Salt

DIRECTIONS:
1. Add oil into the inner pot of instant pot and set the pot on sauté mode. Add onion and chicken and cook for 5 minutes. Add rice, oregano, lemon juice, garlic, broth, pepper, and salt and stir everything well.
2. Seal pot with lid and cook on high for 4 minutes. Once done, release pressure using quick release. Remove lid. Add parsley, zucchini, and bell peppers and stir well.

3. Seal pot again with lid and select manual and set timer for 5 minutes. Release pressure using quick release. Remove lid. Stir well and serve.

NUTRITION: Calories 500 Fat 16.5 g Carbohydrates 48 g Protein 38.7 g

Flavorful Chicken Tacos

Preparation Time: 10 minutes

Cooking Time: 10 minutes

Servings: 3

INGREDIENTS:
- 2 chicken breasts, skinless and boneless
- 1 tbsp chili powder
- 1/2 tsp ground cumin
- 1/2 tsp garlic powder
- 1/4 tsp onion powder
- 1/2 tsp paprika
- 4 oz can green chilis, diced
- 1/4 cup chicken broth
- 14 oz can tomato, diced
- Pepper
- Salt

DIRECTIONS:
1. Add all ingredients except chicken into the instant pot and stir well. Add chicken and stir. Seal pot with lid and cook on high for 10 minutes.
2. Once done, allow to release pressure naturally for 5 minutes then release remaining using quick release. Remove lid.
3. Remove chicken from pot and shred using a fork. Return shredded chicken to the pot and stir well. Serve and enjoy.

NUTRITION: Calories 237 Fat 8 g Carbohydrates 10.8 g Protein 30.5 g

Quinoa Chicken Bowls

Preparation Time: 10 minutes

Cooking Time: 6 minutes

Servings: 4

INGREDIENTS:
- 1 lb. chicken breasts, skinless, boneless, and cut into chunks
- 14 oz can chickpeas, drained and rinsed
- 1 cup olives, pitted and sliced
- 1 cup cherry tomatoes, halved
- 1 cucumber, sliced
- 2 tsp Greek seasoning
- 1 1/2 cups chicken broth
- 1 cup quinoa, rinsed and drained
- Pepper
- Salt

DIRECTIONS:
1. Add broth and quinoa into the instant pot and stir well. Season chicken with Greek seasoning, pepper, and salt and place into the instant pot.
2. Seal pot with lid and cook on high for 6 minutes. Once done, release pressure using quick release. Remove lid. Stir quinoa and chicken mixture well.
3. Add remaining ingredients and stir everything well. Serve immediately and enjoy it.

NUTRITION: Calories 566 Fat 16.4 g Carbohydrates 57.4 g Protein 46.8 g

Quick Chicken with Mushrooms

Preparation Time: 10 minutes

Cooking Time: 22 minutes

Servings: 6

INGREDIENTS:
- 2 lb. chicken breasts, skinless and boneless
- 1/2 cup heavy cream
- 1/3 cup water
- 3/4 lb. mushrooms, sliced
- 3 tbsp olive oil
- 1 tsp Italian seasoning
- Pepper
- Salt

DIRECTIONS:
1. Add oil into the inner pot of instant pot and set the pot on sauté mode. Season chicken with Italian seasoning, pepper, and salt.
2. Add chicken to the pot and sauté for 5 minutes. Remove chicken from pot and set aside. Add mushrooms and sauté for 5 minutes or until mushrooms are lightly brown.
3. Return chicken to the pot. Add water and stir well. Seal pot with a lid and select manual and set timer for 12 minutes.
4. Once done, release pressure using quick release. Remove lid. Remove chicken from pot and place on a plate.
5. Set pot on sauté mode. Add heavy cream and stir well and cook for 5 minutes. Pour

mushroom sauce over chicken and serve.
NUTRITION: Calories 396 Fat 22.3 g Carbohydrates
2.2 g Protein 45.7 g

Herb Garlic Chicken

Preparation Time: 10 minutes

Cooking Time: 12 minutes

Servings: 8

INGREDIENTS:
- 4 lb. chicken breasts, skinless and boneless
- 1 tbsp garlic powder
- 2 tbsp dried Italian herb mix
- 2 tbsp olive oil
- 1/4 cup chicken stock
- Pepper
- Salt

DIRECTIONS:
1. Coat chicken with oil and season with dried herb, garlic powder, pepper, and salt. Place chicken into the instant pot. Pour stock over the chicken. Seal pot with a lid and select manual and set timer for 12 minutes.
2. Once done, allow to release pressure naturally for 5 minutes then release remaining using quick release. Remove lid. Shred chicken using a fork and serve.

NUTRITION: Calories 502 Fat 20.8 g Carbohydrates 7.8 g Protein 66.8 g

Flavorful Mediterranean Chicken

Preparation Time: 10 minutes

Cooking Time: 20 minutes

Servings: 8

INGREDIENTS:
- 2 lb. chicken thighs
- 1/2 cup olives
- 28 oz can tomato, diced
- 1 1/2 tsp dried oregano
- 2 tsp dried parsley
- 1/2 tsp ground coriander powder
- 1/4 tsp chili pepper
- 1 tsp onion powder
- 1 tsp paprika
- 2 cups onion, chopped
- 2 tbsp olive oil
- Pepper
- Salt

DIRECTIONS:
1. Add oil into the inner pot of instant pot and set the pot on sauté mode. Add chicken and cook until browned. Transfer chicken on a plate. Add onion and sauté for 5 minutes.
2. Add all spices, tomatoes, and salt and cook for 2-3 minutes. Return chicken to the pot and stir everything well. Seal pot with lid and cook on high for 8 minutes.
3. Once done, release pressure using quick release. Remove lid. Add olives and stir

well. Serve and enjoy.
NUTRITION: Calories 292 Fat 13 g Carbohydrates
8.9 g Protein 34.3 g

Artichoke Olive Chicken

Preparation Time: 10 minutes

Cooking Time: 8 minutes

Servings: 6

INGREDIENTS:
- 2 1/2 lb. chicken breasts, skinless and boneless
- 14 oz can artichokes
- 1/2 cup olives, pitted
- 3/4 cup prunes
- 1 tbsp capers
- 1 1/2 tbsp garlic, chopped
- 3 tbsp red wine vinegar
- 2 tsp dried oregano
- 1/3 cup wine
- Pepper
- Salt

DIRECTIONS:
1. Add all ingredients except chicken into the instant pot and stir well. Add chicken and mix well. Seal pot with lid and cook on high for 8 minutes.
2. Once done, allow to release pressure naturally for 10 minutes then release remaining using quick release. Remove lid. Serve and enjoy.

NUTRITION: Calories 472 Fat 15.5 g Carbohydrates 22.7 g Protein 57.6 g

Easy Chicken Piccata

Preparation Time: 10 minutes

Cooking Time: 41 minutes

Servings: 6

INGREDIENTS:
- 8 chicken thighs, bone-in, and skin-on
- 2 tbsp fresh parsley, chopped
- 1 tbsp olive oil
- 3 tbsp capers
- 2 tbsp fresh lemon juice
- 1/2 cup chicken broth
- 1/4 cup dry white wine
- 1 tbsp garlic, minced

DIRECTIONS:
1. Add oil into the inner pot of instant pot and set the pot on sauté mode. Add garlic and sauté for 1 minute. Add wine and cook for 5 minutes or until wine reduced by half.
2. Add lemon juice and broth and stir well. Add chicken and seal pot with the lid and select manual and set a timer for 30 minutes.
3. Once done, release pressure using quick release. Remove lid. Remove chicken from pot and place on a baking tray. Broil chicken for 5 minutes. Add capers and stir well. Garnish with parsley and serve.

NUTRITION: Calories 406 Fat 17 g Carbohydrates 1.2 g Protein 57 g

Garlic Thyme Chicken Drumsticks

Preparation Time: 10 minutes

Cooking Time: 18 minutes

Servings: 4

INGREDIENTS:
- 8 chicken drumsticks, skin-on
- 2 tbsp balsamic vinegar
- 2/3 cup can tomato, diced
- 6 garlic cloves
- 1 tsp lemon zest, grated
- 1 tsp dried thyme
- 1/4 tsp red pepper flakes
- 1 1/2 onions, cut into wedges
- 1 tbsp olive oil
- Pepper
- Salt

DIRECTIONS:
1. Add oil into the inner pot of instant pot and set the pot on sauté mode. Add onion and 1/2 tsp salt and sauté for 2-3 minutes.
2. Add chicken, garlic, lemon zest, red pepper flakes, and thyme and mix well. Add vinegar and tomatoes and stir well.
3. Seal pot with lid and cook on high for 15 minutes. Once done, release pressure using quick release. Remove lid. Stir well and serve.

NUTRITION: Calories 220 Fat 8.9 g Carbohydrates 7.8 g Protein 26.4 g

Tender Chicken & Mushrooms

Preparation Time: 10 minutes

Cooking Time: 21 minutes

Servings: 6

INGREDIENTS:
- 1 lb. chicken breasts, skinless, boneless, & cut into 1-inch pieces
- 1/4 cup olives, sliced
- 2 oz feta cheese, crumbled
- 1/4 cup sherry
- 1 cup chicken broth
- 1 tsp Italian seasoning
- 12 oz mushrooms, sliced
- 2 celery stalks, diced
- 1 tsp garlic, minced
- 1/2 cup onion, chopped
- 2 tbsp olive oil
- Pepper
- Salt

DIRECTIONS:
1. Add oil into the inner pot of instant pot and set the pot on sauté mode. Add mushrooms, celery, garlic, and onion and sauté for 5-7 minutes.
2. Add chicken, Italian seasoning, pepper, and salt and stir well and cook for 4 minutes. Add sherry and broth and stir well. Seal pot with lid and cook on high for 10 minutes.

3. Once done, allow to release pressure naturally for 10 minutes then release remaining using quick release. Remove lid. Add olives and feta cheese and stir well. Serve and enjoy.

NUTRITION: Calories 244 Fat 13.5 g Carbohydrates 4.1 g Protein 26 g

Delicious Chicken Casserole

Preparation Time: 10 minutes

Cooking Time: 20 minutes

Servings: 4

INGREDIENTS:
- 1 lb. chicken breasts, skinless, boneless, & cubed
- 2 tsp paprika
- 3 tbsp tomato paste
- 1 cup chicken stock
- 4 tomatoes, chopped
- 1 small eggplant, chopped
- 1 tbsp Italian seasoning
- 2 bell pepper, sliced
- 1 onion, sliced
- 1 tbsp garlic, minced
- 1 tbsp olive oil
- Pepper
- Salt

DIRECTIONS:
1. Add oil into the inner pot of instant pot and set the pot on sauté mode. Season chicken with pepper and salt and add into the instant pot. Cook chicken until lightly golden brown.
2. Remove chicken from pot and place on a plate. Add garlic and onion and sauté until onion is softened about 3-5 minutes.
3. Return chicken to the pot. Pour remaining ingredients over chicken and stir well. Seal

pot with lid and cook on high for 10 minutes.

4. Once done, release pressure using quick release. Remove lid. Stir well and serve.

NUTRITION: Calories 356 Fat 13.9 g Carbohydrates 22.7 g Protein 36.9 g

Perfect Chicken & Rice

Preparation Time: 10 minutes

Cooking Time: 25 minutes

Servings: 4

INGREDIENTS:
- 1 lb. chicken breasts, skinless and boneless
- 1 tsp olive oil
- 1 cup onion, diced
- 1 tsp garlic minced
- 4 carrots, peeled and sliced
- 1 tbsp Mediterranean spice mix
- 2 cups brown rice, rinsed
- 2 cups chicken stock
- Pepper
- Salt

DIRECTIONS:
1. Add oil into the inner pot of instant pot and set the pot on sauté mode. Add garlic and onion and sauté until onion is softened.
2. Add stock, carrot, rice, and Mediterranean spice mix and stir well. Place chicken on top of rice mixture and season with pepper and salt. Do not mix.
3. Seal pot with a lid and select manual and set timer for 20 minutes. Once done, allow to release pressure naturally for 10 minutes then release remaining using quick release. Remove lid.
4. Remove chicken from pot and shred using a fork. Return shredded chicken to the pot and stir well. Serve and enjoy.

NUTRITION: Calories 612 Fat 12.4 g Carbohydrates 81.7 g Protein 41.1 g

Moroccan Chicken

Preparation Time: 10 minutes

Cooking Time: 25 minutes

Servings: 6

INGREDIENTS:
- 2 lb. chicken breasts, cut into chunks
- 1/2 tsp cinnamon
- 1 tsp turmeric
- 1/2 tsp ginger
- 1 tsp cumin
- 2 tbsp Dijon mustard
- 1 tbsp molasses
- 1 tbsp honey
- 2 tbsp tomato paste
- 5 garlic cloves, chopped
- 2 onions, cut into quarters
- 2 green bell peppers, cut into strips
- 2 red bell peppers, cut into strips
- 2 cups olives, pitted
- 1 lemon, peeled and sliced
- 2 tbsp olive oil
- Pepper
- Salt

DIRECTIONS:
1. Add oil into the inner pot of instant pot and set the pot on sauté mode. Add chicken and sauté for 5 minutes. Add remaining ingredients and stir everything well.
2. Seal pot with a lid and select manual and set timer for 20 minutes. Once done, release pressure using quick release.

Remove lid. Stir well and serve.
NUTRITION: Calories 446 Fat 21.2 g Carbohydrates
18.5 g Protein 45.8 g

Flavorful Cafe Rio Chicken

Preparation Time: 10 minutes

Cooking Time: 12 minutes

Servings: 6

INGREDIENTS:
- 2 lb. chicken breasts, skinless and boneless
- 1/2 cup chicken stock
- 2 1/2 tbsp ranch seasoning
- 1/2 tbsp ground cumin
- 1/2 tbsp chili powder
- 1/2 tbsp garlic, minced
- 2/3 cup Italian dressing
- Pepper
- Salt

DIRECTIONS:
1. Add chicken into the instant pot. Mix together remaining ingredients and pour over chicken. Seal pot with a lid and select manual and set timer for 12 minutes.
2. Once done, allow to release pressure naturally for 10 minutes then release remaining using quick release. Remove lid. Shred the chicken using a fork and serve.

NUTRITION: Calories 382 Fat 18.9 g Carbohydrates 3.6 g Protein 44.1 g

Zesty Veggie Chicken

Preparation Time: 10 minutes

Cooking Time: 5 minutes

Servings: 4

INGREDIENTS:
- 1 lb. chicken tender, skinless, boneless and cut into chunks
- 10 oz of frozen vegetables
- 1/3 cup zesty Italian dressing
- 1/2 tsp Italian seasoning
- 1 cup fried onions
- 2/3 cup rice
- 1 cup chicken broth
- Pepper
- Salt

DIRECTIONS:
1. Add all ingredients except vegetables into the instant pot. Meanwhile, cook frozen vegetables in microwave according to packet instructions.
2. Seal pot with lid and cook on high for 5 minutes. Once done, allow to release pressure naturally for 10 minutes then release remaining using quick release. Remove lid.
3. Add cooked vegetables and stir well. Serve and enjoy.

NUTRITION: Calories 482 Fat 15.9 g Carbohydrates 40.5 g Protein 38.3 g

Cilantro Lemon Shrimp

Preparation time: 20 minutes

Cooking time: 10 minutes

Servings: 4

INGREDIENTS:
- 1/3 cup lemon juice
- 4 garlic cloves
- 1 cup fresh cilantro leaves
- ½ teaspoon ground coriander
- 3 tablespoons extra-virgin olive oil
- 1 teaspoon salt
- 1½ pounds (680 g) large shrimp (21 to 25), deveined and shells removed

DIRECTIONS:
1. In a food processor, pulse the lemon juice, garlic, cilantro, coriander, olive oil, and salt 10 times. Put the shrimp in a bowl or plastic zip-top bag, pour in the cilantro marinade, and let sit for 15 minutes.
2. Preheat a skillet on high heat. Put the shrimp and marinade in the skillet. Cook the shrimp for 3 minutes on each side. Serve warm.

NUTRITION: Calories: 225 Fat: 12g Protein: 28g Carbs: 5g

Seafood Risotto

Preparation time: 15 minutes

Cooking time: 30 minutes

Servings: 4

INGREDIENTS:
- 6 cups vegetable broth
- 3 tablespoons extra-virgin olive oil
- 1 large onion, chopped
- 3 cloves garlic, minced
- ½ teaspoon saffron threads
- 1½ cups arborio rice
- 1½ teaspoons salt
- 8 ounces (227 g) shrimp (21 to 25), peeled and deveined
- 8 ounces (227 g) scallops

DIRECTIONS:
1. In a large saucepan over medium heat, bring the broth to a low simmer. In a large skillet over medium heat, cook the olive oil, onion, garlic, and saffron for 3 minutes.
2. Add the rice, salt, and 1 cup of the broth to the skillet. Stir the ingredients together and cook over low heat until most of the liquid is absorbed.
3. Repeat steps with broth, adding ½ cup of broth at a time, and cook until all but ½ cup of the broth is absorbed.
4. Add the shrimp and scallops when you stir in the final ½ cup of broth. Cover and let cook for 10 minutes. Serve warm.

NUTRITION: Calories: 460 Fat: 12g Protein: 24g Carbs: 64g

Garlic Shrimp Black Bean Pasta

Preparation time: 15 minutes

Cooking time: 15 minutes

Servings: 4

INGREDIENTS:
- 1 pound (454 g) black bean linguine or spaghetti
- 1 pound (454 g) fresh shrimp, peeled and deveined
- 4 tablespoons extra-virgin olive oil
- 1 onion, finely chopped
- 3 garlic cloves, minced
- ¼ cup basil, cut into strips

DIRECTIONS:
1. Bring a large pot of water to a boil and cook the pasta according to the package instructions.
2. In the last 5 minutes of cooking the pasta, add the shrimp to the hot water and allow them to cook for 3 to 5 minutes.
3. Once they turn pink, take them out of the hot water, and, if you think you may have overcooked them, run them under cool water. Set aside.
4. Reserve 1 cup of the pasta cooking water and drain the noodles. In the same pan, heat the oil over medium-high heat and cook the onion and garlic for 7 to 10 minutes.

5. Once the onion is translucent, add the pasta back in and toss well. Plate the pasta, then top with shrimp and garnish with basil.

NUTRITION: Calories: 668 Fat: 19g Protein: 57g Carbs: 73g

Fast Seafood Paella

Preparation time: 15 minutes

Cooking time: 20 minutes

Servings: 4

INGREDIENTS:
- ¼ cup plus 1 tablespoon extra-virgin olive oil
- 1 large onion, finely chopped
- 2 tomatoes, peeled and chopped
- 1½ tablespoons garlic powder
- 1½ cups medium-grain Spanish paella rice or arborio rice
- 2 carrots, finely diced
- Salt, to taste
- 1 tablespoon sweet paprika
- 8 ounces (227 g) lobster meat or canned crab
- ½ cup frozen peas
- 3 cups chicken stock, plus more if needed
- 1 cup dry white wine
- 6 jumbo shrimp, unpeeled

- $1/_3$ pound (136 g) calamari rings

- 1 lemon, halved

DIRECTIONS:
1. In a large sauté pan or skillet (16-inch is ideal), heat the oil over medium heat until small bubbles start to escape from oil.

2. Add the onion and cook for about 3 minutes, until fragrant, then add tomatoes and garlic powder. Cook for 5 to 10 minutes, until the tomatoes are reduced by half and the consistency is sticky.
3. Stir in the rice, carrots, salt, paprika, lobster, and peas and mix well. In a pot or microwave-safe bowl, heat the chicken stock to almost boiling, then add it to the rice mixture. Bring to a simmer, then add the wine.
4. Smooth out the rice in the bottom of the pan. Cover and cook on low for 10 minutes, mixing occasionally, to prevent burning.
5. Top the rice with the shrimp, cover, and cook for 5 more minutes. Add additional broth to the pan if the rice looks dried out.
6. Right before removing the skillet from the heat, add the calamari rings. Toss the ingredients frequently.
7. In about 2 minutes, the rings will look opaque. Remove the pan from the heat immediately—you don't want the paella to overcook). Squeeze fresh lemon juice over the dish.

NUTRITION: Calories: 632 Fat: 20g Protein: 34g Carbs: 71g

Crispy Fried Sardines

Preparation time: 15 minutes

Cooking time: 5 minutes

Servings: 4

INGREDIENTS:
- Avocado oil, as needed
- 1½ pounds (680 g) whole fresh sardines, scales removed
- 1 teaspoon salt
- 1 teaspoon freshly ground black pepper
- 2 cups flour

DIRECTIONS:
1. Preheat a deep skillet over medium heat. Pour in enough oil so there is about 1 inch of it in the pan. Season the fish with the salt and pepper.
2. Dredge the fish in the flour so it is completely covered. Slowly drop in 1 fish at a time, making sure not to overcrowd the pan.
3. Cook for about 3 minutes on each side or just until the fish begins to brown on all sides. Serve warm.

NUTRITION: Calories: 794 Fat: 47g Protein: 48g Carbs: 44g

Orange Roasted Salmon

Preparation time: 15 minutes
Cooking time : 25 minutes

Servings: 4

INGREDIENTS:
- ½ cup extra-virgin olive oil, divided
- 2 tablespoons balsamic vinegar
- 2 tablespoons garlic powder, divided
- 1 tablespoon cumin seeds
- 1 teaspoon sea salt, divided
- 1 teaspoon freshly ground black pepper, divided
- 2 teaspoons smoked paprika
- 4 (8-ounce / 227-g) salmon fillets, skinless
- 2 small red onion, thinly sliced
- ½ cup halved Campari tomatoes
- 1 small fennel bulb, thinly sliced lengthwise
- 1 large carrot, thinly sliced
- 8 medium portobello mushrooms
- 8 medium radishes, sliced ⅛ inch thick
- ½ cup dry white wine
- ½ lime, zested
- Handful cilantro leaves
- ½ cup halved pitted Kalamata olives
- 1 orange, thinly sliced
- 4 roasted sweet potatoes, cut in wedges lengthwise

DIRECTIONS:
1. Preheat the oven to 375ºF (190ºC). In a medium bowl, mix 6 tablespoons of olive oil, the balsamic vinegar, 1 tablespoon of garlic powder, the cumin seeds, ¼

teaspoon of sea salt, ¼ teaspoon of pepper, and the paprika.
2. Put the salmon in the bowl and marinate while preparing the vegetables, about 10 minutes.
3. Heat an oven-safe sauté pan or skillet on medium-high heat and sear the top of the salmon for about 2 minutes, or until lightly brown. Set aside.
4. Add the remaining 2 tablespoons of olive oil to the same skillet. Once it's hot, add the onion, tomatoes, fennel, carrot, mushrooms, radishes, the remaining 1 teaspoon of garlic powder, ¾ teaspoon of salt, and ¾ teaspoon of pepper.
5. Mix well and cook for 5 to 7 minutes, until fragrant. Add wine and mix well. Place the salmon on top of the vegetable mixture, browned-side up.
6. Sprinkle the fish with lime zest and cilantro and place the olives around the fish. Put orange slices over the fish and cook for about 7 additional minutes.
7. While this is baking, add the sliced sweet potato wedges on a baking sheet and bake this alongside the skillet. Remove from the oven, cover the skillet tightly, and let rest for about 3 minutes.

NUTRITION: Calories: 841 Fat: 41g Protein: 59g Carbs: 60g

Lemon Rosemary Branzino

Preparation time: 15 minutes

Cooking time: 30 minutes

Servings: 4

INGREDIENTS:
- 4 tablespoons extra-virgin olive oil, divided
- 2 (8-ounce / 227-g) branzino fillets, preferably at least 1 inch thick
- 1 garlic clove, minced
- 1 bunch scallions, white part only, thinly sliced
- ½ cup sliced pitted Kalamata or other good -quality black olives
- 1 large carrot, cut into ¼-inch rounds
- 10 to 12 small cherry tomatoes, halved
- ½ cup dry white wine
- 2 tablespoons paprika
- 2 teaspoons kosher salt
- ½ tablespoon ground chili pepper, preferably Turkish or Aleppo
- 2 rosemary sprigs or 1 tablespoon dried rosemary
- 1 small lemon, very thinly sliced

DIRECTIONS:
1. Warm a large, oven-safe sauté pan or skillet over high heat until hot, about 2 minutes. Carefully add 1 tablespoon of olive oil and heat until it shimmers, 10 to 15 seconds.

2. Brown the branzino fillets for 2 minutes, skin-side up. Carefully flip the fillets skin-side down and cook for another 2 minutes, until browned. Set aside.
3. Swirl 2 tablespoons of olive oil around the skillet to coat evenly. Add the garlic, scallions, kalamata olives, carrot, and tomatoes, and let the vegetables sauté for 5 minutes, until softened.
4. Add the wine, stirring until all ingredients are well integrated. Carefully place the fish over the sauce. Preheat the oven to 450°F (235°C).
5. While the oven is heating, brush the fillets with 1 tablespoon of olive oil and season with paprika, salt, and chili pepper.
6. Top each fillet with a rosemary sprig and several slices of lemon. Scatter the olives over fish and around the pan. Roast until lemon slices are browned or singed, about 10 minutes.

NUTRITION: calories: 725 fat: 43g protein: 58g carbs: 25g

Almond-Crusted Swordfish

Preparation time: 15 minutes

Cooking time: 15 minutes

Servings: 4

INGREDIENTS:
- ½ cup almond flour
- ¼ cup crushed Marcona almonds
- ½ to 1 teaspoon salt, divided
- 2 pounds (907 g) Swordfish, preferably 1 inch thick
- 1 large egg, beaten (optional)
- ¼ cup pure apple cider
- ¼ cup extra-virgin olive oil, plus more for frying
- 3 to 4 sprigs flat-leaf parsley, chopped
- 1 lemon, juiced
- 1 tablespoon Spanish paprika
- 5 medium baby portobello mushrooms, chopped (optional)
- 4 or 5 chopped scallions, both green and white parts
- 3 to 4 garlic cloves, peeled
- ¼ cup chopped pitted Kalamata olives

DIRECTIONS:
1. On a dinner plate, spread the flour and crushed Marcona almonds and mix in the salt. Alternately, pour the flour, almonds, and ¼ teaspoon of salt into a large plastic food storage bag.

2. Add the fish and coat it with the flour mixture. If a thicker coat is desired, repeat this step after dipping the fish in the egg (if using).
3. In a measuring cup, combine the apple cider, ¼ cup of olive oil, parsley, lemon juice, paprika, and ¼ teaspoon of salt. Mix well and set aside.
4. In a large, heavy-bottom sauté pan or skillet, pour the olive oil to a depth of ⅛ inch and heat on medium heat.
5. Once the oil is hot, add the fish and brown for 3 to 5 minutes, then turn the fish over and add the mushrooms (If using), scallions, garlic, and olives.
6. Cook for an additional 3 minutes. Once the other side of the fish is brown, remove the fish from the pan and set aside.
7. Pour the cider mixture into the skillet and mix well with the vegetables. Put the fried fish into the skillet on top of the mixture and cook with sauce on medium-low heat for 10 minutes, until the fish flakes easily with a fork.
8. Carefully remove the fish from the pan and plate. Spoon the sauce over the fish. Serve with white rice or home-fried potatoes.

NUTRITION: Calories: 620 Fat: 37g Protein: 63g Carbs: 10g

Sea Bass Crusted with Moroccan Spices

Preparation time: 15 minutes

Cooking time: 40 minutes

Servings: 4

INGREDIENTS:
- 1½ teaspoons ground turmeric, divided
- ¾ teaspoon saffron
- ½ teaspoon ground cumin
- ¼ teaspoon kosher salt
- ¼ teaspoon freshly ground black pepper
- 1½ pounds (680 g) sea bass fillets, about ½ inch thick
- 8 tablespoons extra-virgin olive oil, divided
- 8 garlic cloves, divided (4 minced cloves and 4 sliced)
- 6 medium baby portobello mushrooms, chopped
- 1 large carrot, sliced on an angle
- 2 sun-dried tomatoes, thinly sliced (optional)
- 2 tablespoons tomato paste
- 1 (15-ounce / 425-g) can chickpeas, drained and rinsed
- 1½ cups low-sodium vegetable broth
- ¼ cup white wine
- 1 tablespoon ground coriander (optional)
- 1 cup sliced artichoke hearts marinated in olive oil
- ½ cup pitted Kalamata olives
- ½ lemon, juiced

- ½ lemon, cut into thin rounds
- 4 to 5 rosemary sprigs or 2 tablespoons dried rosemary
- Fresh cilantro, for garnish

DIRECTIONS:

1. In a small mixing bowl, combine 1 teaspoon turmeric and the saffron and cumin. Season with salt and pepper. Season both sides of the fish with the spice mixture.
2. Add 3 tablespoons of olive oil and work the fish to make sure it's well coated with the spices and the olive oil.
3. In a large sauté pan or skillet, heat 2 tablespoons of olive oil over medium heat until shimmering but not smoking. Sear the top side of the sea bass for about 1 minute, or until golden. Remove and set aside.
4. In the same skillet, add the minced garlic and cook very briefly, tossing regularly, until fragrant. Add the mushrooms, carrot, sun-dried tomatoes (if using), and tomato paste.
5. Cook for 3 to 4 minutes over medium heat, tossing frequently, until fragrant. Add the chickpeas, broth, wine, coriander (if using), and the sliced garlic.
6. Stir in the remaining ½ teaspoon ground turmeric. Raise the heat, if needed, and bring to a boil, then lower heat to simmer. Cover part of the way and let the sauce simmer for about 20 minutes, until thickened.

7. Carefully add the seared fish to the skillet. Ladle a bit of the sauce on top of the fish. Add the artichokes, olives, lemon juice and slices, and rosemary sprigs.
8. Cook another 10 minutes or until the fish is fully cooked and flaky. Garnish with fresh cilantro.

NUTRITION: Calories: 696 Fat: 41g Protein: 48g Carbs: 37g

Shrimp with Garlic and Mushrooms

Preparation time: 15 minutes

Cooking time: 15 minutes

Servings: 4

INGREDIENTS:
- 1 pound (454 g) peeled and deveined fresh shrimp
- 1 teaspoon salt
- 1 cup extra-virgin olive oil
- 8 large garlic cloves, thinly sliced
- 4 ounces (113 g) sliced mushrooms (shiitake, baby bella, or button)
- ½ teaspoon red pepper flakes
- ¼ cup chopped fresh flat-leaf Italian parsley
- Zucchini noodles or riced cauliflower, for serving

DIRECTIONS:
1. Rinse the shrimp and pat dry. Place in a small bowl and sprinkle with the salt. In a large rimmed, thick skillet, heat the olive oil over medium-low heat.
2. Add the garlic and heat until very fragrant, 3 to 4 minutes, reducing the heat if the garlic starts to burn.
3. Add the mushrooms and sauté for 5 minutes, until softened. Add the shrimp and red pepper flakes and sauté until the shrimp begins to turn pink, another 3 to 4 minutes.

4. Remove from the heat and stir in the parsley. Serve over zucchini noodles or riced cauliflower.

NUTRITION: Calories: 620 Fat: 56g Protein: 24g Carbs: 4g

Pistachio-Crusted Whitefish

Preparation Time: 10 minutes

Cooking Time: 20 minutes

Servings: 2

INGREDIENTS:
- ¼ cup shelled pistachios
- 1 tablespoon fresh parsley
- 1 tablespoon grated Parmesan cheese
- 1 tablespoon panko bread crumbs
- 2 tablespoons olive oil
- ¼ teaspoon salt
- 10 ounces skinless whitefish (1 large piece or 2 smaller ones)

DIRECTIONS:
1. Preheat the oven to 350°F and set the rack to the middle position. Line a sheet pan with foil or parchment paper.
2. Combine all of the ingredients except the fish in a mini food processor, and pulse until the nuts are finely ground.
3. Alternatively, you can mince the nuts with a chef's knife and combine the ingredients by hand in a small bowl.
4. Place the fish on the sheet pan. Spread the nut mixture evenly over the fish and pat it down lightly.
5. Bake the fish for 20 to 30 minutes, depending on the thickness, until it flakes easily with a fork.

6. Keep in mind that a thicker cut of fish takes a bit longer to bake. You'll know it's done when it's opaque, flakes apart easily with a fork, or reaches an internal temperature of 145°F

NUTRITION: Calories – 185, Carbs - 23.8 g, Protein - 10.1 g, Fat - 5.2 g

Crispy Homemade Fish Sticks Recipe

Preparation Time: 10 minutes

Cooking Time: 15 minutes

Servings: 2

INGREDIENTS:
- ½ cup of flour
- 1 beaten egg
- 1 cup of flour
- ½ cup of parmesan cheese
- ½ cup of bread crumbs.
- Zest of 1 lemon juice
- Parsley
- Salt
- 1 teaspoon of black pepper
- 1 tablespoon of sweet paprika
- 1 teaspoon of oregano
- 1 ½ lb. of salmon
- Extra virgin olive oil

DIRECTIONS:
1. Preheat your oven to about 450 degrees F. Get a bowl, dry your salmon and season its two sides with the salt.
2. Then chop into small sizes of 1½ inch length each. Get a bowl and mix black pepper with oregano.
3. Add paprika to the mixture and blend it. Then spice the fish stick with the mixture you have just made. Get another dish and pour your flours.

4. You will need a different bowl again to pour your egg wash into. Pick yet the fourth dish, mix your breadcrumb with your parmesan and add lemon zest to the mixture.
5. Return to the fish sticks and dip each fish into flour such that both sides are coated with flour. As you dip each fish into flour, take it out and dip it into egg wash and lastly, dip it in the breadcrumb mixture.
6. Do this for all fish sticks and arrange on a baking sheet. Ensure you oil the baking sheet before arranging the stick thereon and drizzle the top of the fish sticks with extra virgin olive oil.
7. Caution: allow excess flours to fall off a fish before dipping it into other ingredients.
8. Also ensure that you do not let the coating peel while you add extra virgin olive oil on top of the fishes.
9. Fix the baking sheet in the middle of the oven and allow it to cook for 13 min. By then, the fishes should be golden brown and you can collect them from the oven, and you can serve immediately.
10. Top it with your lemon zest, parsley and fresh lemon juice.

NUTRITION: 119 Cal, 3.4g of fat, 293.1mg of sodium, 9.3g of carbs, 13.5g of protein.

Sauced Shellfish in White Wine

Preparation Time: 10 minutes

Cooking Time: 10 minutes

Servings: 2

INGREDIENTS:
- 2-lbs fresh cuttlefish
- ½-cup olive oil
- 1-pc large onion, finely chopped
- 1-cup of Robola white wine
- ¼-cup lukewarm water
- 1-pc bay leaf
- ½-bunch parsley, chopped
- 4-pcs tomatoes, grated
- Salt and pepper

DIRECTIONS:
1. Take out the hard centerpiece of cartilage (cuttlebone), the bag of ink, and the intestines from the cuttlefish.
2. Wash the cleaned cuttlefish with running water. Slice it into small pieces, and drain excess water.
3. Heat the oil in a saucepan placed over medium-high heat and sauté the onion for 3 minutes until tender.
4. Add the sliced cuttlefish and pour in the white wine. Cook for 5 minutes until it simmers.
5. Pour in the water, and add the tomatoes, bay leaf, parsley, tomatoes, salt, and pepper. Simmer the mixture over low heat

until the cuttlefish slices are tender and left with their thick sauce. Serve them warm with rice.

6. Be careful not to overcook the cuttlefish as its texture becomes very hard. A safe rule of thumb is grilling the cuttlefish over a ragingly hot fire for 3 minutes before using it in any recipe.

NUTRITION: Calories: 308, Fats: 18.1g, Dietary Fiber: 1.5g, Carbohydrates: 8g, Protein: 25.6g

Pistachio Sole Fish

Preparation Time : 5 minutes

Cooking Time: 10 minutes

Servings: 2

INGREDIENTS:
- 4 (5 ounces) boneless sole fillets
- ½ cup pistachios, finely chopped
- Juice of 1 lemon
- teaspoon extra virgin olive oil

DIRECTIONS:
1. Pre-heat your oven to 350 degrees Fahrenheit
2. Wrap baking sheet using parchment paper and keep it on the side
3. Pat fish dry with kitchen towels and lightly season with salt and pepper
4. Take a small bowl and stir in pistachios
5. Place sol on the prepped sheet and press 2 tablespoons of pistachio mixture on top of each fillet
6. Rub the fish with lemon juice and olive oil
7. Bake for 10 minutes until the top is golden and fish flakes with a fork

NUTRITION: 166 Calories 6g Fat 2g Carbohydrates

Speedy Tilapia with Red Onion and Avocado

Preparation time: 10 minutes

Cooking time: 5 minutes

Servings : 2

INGREDIENTS:
- 1 tablespoon extra-virgin olive oil
- 1 tablespoon freshly squeezed orange juice
- ¼ teaspoon kosher or sea salt
- 4 (4-ounces) tilapia fillets, more oblong than square, skin-on or skinned
- ¼ cup chopped red onion (about 1/8 onion)
- 1 avocado, pitted, skinned, and sliced

DIRECTIONS:
1. In a 9-inch glass pie dish, use a fork to mix together the oil, orange juice, and salt. Working with one fillet at a time, place each in the pie dish and turn to coat on all sides.
2. Arrange the fillets in a wagon-wheel formation, so that one end of each fillet is in the center of the dish and the other end is temporarily draped over the edge of the dish.
3. Top each fillet with 1 tablespoon of onion, then fold the end of the fillet that's hanging over the edge in half over the onion.
4. When finished, you should have 4 folded-over fillets with the fold against the outer edge of the dish and the ends all in the

center.
5. Cover the dish with plastic wrap, leaving a small part open at the edge to vent the steam. Microwave on high for about 3 minutes.
6. The fish is done when it just begins to separate into flakes (chunks) when pressed gently with a fork. Top the fillets with the avocado and serve.

NUTRITION: 4 g carbohydrates, 3 g fiber, 22 g protein

Steamed Mussels in white Wine Sauce

Preparation time: 5 minutes

Cooking time: 10 minutes

Servings: 2

INGREDIENTS:
- 2 pounds small mussels
- 1 tablespoon extra-virgin olive oil
- 1 cup thinly sliced red onion
- 3 garlic cloves, sliced
- 1 cup dry white wine
- 2 (¼-inch-thick) lemon slices
- ¼ teaspoon freshly ground black pepper
- ¼ teaspoon kosher or sea salt
- Fresh lemon wedges, for serving (optional)

DIRECTIONS:
1. In a large colander in the sink, run cold water over the mussels (but don't let the mussels sit in standing water).
2. All the shells should be closed tight; discard any shells that are a little bit open or any shells that are cracked. Leave the mussels in the colander until you're ready to use them.
3. In a large skillet over medium-high heat, heat the oil. Add the onion and cook for 4 minutes, stirring occasionally.
4. Add the garlic and cook for 1 minute, stirring constantly. Add the wine, lemon slices, pepper, and salt, and bring to a simmer. Cook for 2 minutes.

5. Add the mussels and cover. Cook for 3 minutes, or until the mussels open their shells. Gently shake the pan two or three times while they are cooking.
6. All the shells should now be wide open. Using a slotted spoon, discard any mussels that are still closed. Spoon the opened mussels into a shallow serving bowl, and pour the broth over the top. Serve with additional fresh lemon slices, if desired.

NUTRITION: Calories 22, 7 g total fat, 1 g fiber, 18 g protein

Orange and Garlic Shrimp

Preparation time: 20 minutes

Cooking time: 10 minutes

Servings : 2

INGREDIENTS:
- 1 large orange
- 3 tablespoons extra-virgin olive oil, divided
- 1 tablespoon chopped fresh Rosemary
- 1 tablespoon chopped fresh thyme
- 3 garlic cloves, minced (about 1½ teaspoons)
- ¼ teaspoon freshly ground black pepper
- ¼ teaspoon kosher or sea salt
- 1½ pounds fresh raw shrimp, shells, and tails removed

DIRECTIONS:
1. Zest the entire orange using a citrus grater. In a large zip-top plastic bag, combine the orange zest and 2 tablespoons of oil with the Rosemary, thyme, garlic, pepper, and salt.
2. Add the shrimp, seal the bag, and gently massage the shrimp until all the ingredients are combined and the shrimp is completely covered with the seasonings. Set aside.
3. Heat a grill, grill pan, or a large skillet over medium heat. Brush on or swirl in the remaining 1 tablespoon of oil.
4. Add half the shrimp, and cook for 4 to 6 minutes, or until the shrimp turn pink and white, flipping halfway through if on the

grill or stirring every minute if in a pan. Transfer the shrimp to a large serving bowl.

5. Repeat with the remaining shrimp, and add them to the bowl.
6. While the shrimp cook, peel the orange and cut the flesh into bite-size pieces. Add to the serving bowl, and toss with the cooked shrimp. Serve immediately or refrigerate and serve cold.

NUTRITION: Calories 190, 8 g total fat, 1 g fiber, 24 g protein

Roasted Shrimp-Gnocchi Bake

Preparation time: 10 minutes

Cooking time: 20 minutes

Servings: 2

INGREDIENTS:
- 1 cup chopped fresh tomato
- 2 tablespoons extra-virgin olive oil
- 2 garlic cloves, minced
- ½ teaspoon freshly ground black pepper
- ¼ teaspoon crushed red pepper
- 1 (12-ounces) jar roasted red peppers
- 1-pound fresh raw shrimp, shells and tails removed
- 1-pound frozen gnocchi (not thawed)
- ½ cup cubed feta cheese
- 1/3 cup fresh torn basil leaves

DIRECTIONS:
1. Preheat the oven to 425°F. In a baking dish, mix the tomatoes, oil, garlic, black pepper, and crushed red pepper. Roast in the oven for 10 minutes.
2. Stir in the roasted peppers and shrimp. Roast for 10 more minutes, until the shrimp turn pink and white.
3. While the shrimp cooks, cook the gnocchi on the stovetop according to the package directions.
4. Drain in a colander and keep warm. Remove the dish from the oven. Mix in the cooked gnocchi, feta, and basil, and serve.

NUTRITION: Calories 227, 7 g total fat, 1 g fiber, 20 g protein

Spicy Shrimp Puttanesca

Preparation time: 5 minutes

Cooking time: 15 minutes

Servings: 2

INGREDIENTS:
- 2 tablespoons extra-virgin olive oil
- 3 anchovy fillets, drained and chopped
- 3 garlic cloves, minced
- ½ teaspoon crushed red pepper
- 1 (14.5-ounces) can low-sodium or no-salt -added diced tomatoes, undrained
- 1 (2.25-ounces) can sliced black olives, drained
- 2 tablespoons capers
- 1 tablespoon chopped fresh oregano
- 1-pound fresh raw shrimp, shells and tails removed

DIRECTIONS:
1. In a large skillet over medium heat, heat the oil. Mix in the anchovies, garlic, and crushed red pepper.
2. Cook for 3 minutes, stirring frequently and mashing up the anchovies with a wooden spoon until they have melted into the oil.
3. Stir in the tomatoes with their juices, olives, capers, and oregano. Turn up the heat to medium-high, and bring to a simmer.
4. When the sauce is lightly bubbling, stir in the shrimp. Reduce the heat to medium, and cook the shrimp for 6 to 8 minutes, or until they turn pink and white, stirring

occasionally, and serve.
NUTRITION: Calories 214, 10 g total fat, 2 g fiber, 26 g protein

Baked Cod with Vegetables

Preparation Time: 15 minutes

Cooking Time: 25 minutes

Serving: 2

INGREDIENTS:
- 1 pound (454 g) thick cod fillet, cut into 4 even portions
- ¼ teaspoon onion powder (optional)
- ¼ teaspoon paprika
- 3 tablespoons extra-virgin olive oil
- 4 medium scallions
- ½ cup fresh chopped basil, divided
- 3 tablespoons minced garlic (optional)
- 2 teaspoons salt
- 2 teaspoons freshly ground black pepper
- ¼ teaspoon dry marjoram (optional)
- 6 sun-dried tomato slices
- ½ cup dry white wine
- ½ cup crumbled feta cheese
- 1 (15-ounce / 425-g) can oil-packed artichoke hearts, drained
- 1 lemon, sliced
- 1 cup pitted kalamata olives
- 1 teaspoon capers (optional)
- 4 small red potatoes, quartered

DIRECTION:
1. Set oven to 375ºF (190ºC).
2. Season the fish with paprika and onion powder (if desired).

3. Heat an ovenproof skillet over medium heat and sear the top side of the cod for about 1 minute until golden. Set aside.
4. Heat the olive oil in the same skillet over medium heat. Add the scallions, ¼ cup of basil, garlic (if desired), salt, pepper, marjoram (if desired), tomato slices, and white wine and stir to combine. Boil then removes from heat.
5. Evenly spread the sauce on the bottom of skillet. Place the cod on top of the tomato basil sauce and scatter with feta cheese. Place the artichokes in the skillet and top with the lemon slices.
6. Scatter with the olives, capers (if desired), and the remaining ¼ cup of basil. Pullout from the heat and transfer to the preheated oven. Bake for 15 to 20 minutes
7. Meanwhile, place the quartered potatoes on a baking sheet or wrapped in aluminum foil. Bake in the oven for 15 minutes.
8. Cool for 5 minutes before serving.

NUTRITION: Calories 1168, 60g fat, 64g protein

Slow Cooker Salmon in Foil

Preparation Time: 5 minutes

Cooking Time: 2 hours

Serving: 2

INGREDIENTS:
- 2 (6-ounce / 170-g) salmon fillets
- 1 tablespoon olive oil
- 2 cloves garlic, minced
- ½ tablespoon lime juice
- 1 teaspoon finely chopped fresh parsley
- ¼ teaspoon black pepper

DIRECTION
1. Spread a length of foil onto a work surface and place the salmon fillets in the middle.
2. Blend olive oil, garlic, lime juice, parsley, and black pepper. Brush the mixture over the fillets. Fold the foil over and crimp the sides to make a packet.
3. Place the packet into the slow cooker, cover, and cook on High for 2 hours
4. Serve hot.

NUTRITION: Calories 446, 21g fat, 65g protein

Dill Chutney Salmon

Preparation Time: 5 minutes

Cooking Time: 3 minutes

Serving: 2

INGREDIENTS:
- Chutney:
- ¼ cup fresh dill
- ¼ cup extra virgin olive oil
- Juice from ½ lemon
- Sea salt, to taste
- Fish:
- 2 cups water
- 2 salmon fillets
- Juice from ½ lemon
- ¼ teaspoon paprika
- Salt and freshly ground pepper to taste

DIRECTION:
1. Pulse all the chutney ingredients in a food processor until creamy. Set aside.
2. Add the water and steamer basket to the Instant Pot. Place salmon fillets, skin-side down, on the steamer basket. Drizzle the lemon juice over salmon and sprinkle with the paprika.
3. Secure the lid. Select the Manual mode and set the cooking time for 3 minutes at High Pressure.
4. Once cooking is complete, do a quick pressure release. Carefully open the lid.
5. Season the fillets with pepper and salt to taste. Serve topped with the dill chutney.

NUTRITION: Calories 636, 41g fat, 65g protein

Garlic-Butter Parmesan Salmon and Asparagus

Preparation Time: 10 minutes

Cooking Time: 15 minutes

Serving: 2

INGREDIENTS:
- 2 (6-ounce / 170-g) salmon fillets, skin on and patted dry
- Pink Himalayan salt
- Freshly ground black pepper, to taste
- 1 pound (454 g) fresh asparagus, ends snapped off
- 3 tablespoons almond butter
- 2 garlic cloves, minced
- ¼ cup grated Parmesan cheese

DIRECTION:
1. Prep oven to 400ºF (205ºC). Line a baking sheet with aluminum foil.
2. Season both sides of the salmon fillets.
3. Situate salmon in the middle of the baking sheet and arrange the asparagus around the salmon.
4. Heat the almond butter in a small saucepan over medium heat.
5. Cook minced garlic
6. Drizzle the garlic-butter sauce over the salmon and asparagus and scatter the Parmesan cheese on top.
7. Bake in the preheated oven for about 12 minutes. You can switch the oven to broil at the end of cooking time for about 3

minutes to get a nice char on the asparagus.
8. Let cool for 5 minutes before serving.
NUTRITION: Calories 435, 26g fat, 42g protein

Lemon Rosemary Roasted Branzino

Preparation Time: 15 minutes
Cooking Time : 30 minutes

Serving: 2

INGREDIENTS:
- 4 tablespoons extra-virgin olive oil, divided
- 2 (8-ounce) Branzino fillets
- 1 garlic clove, minced
- 1 bunch scallions
- 10 to 12 small cherry tomatoes, halved
- 1 large carrot, cut into ¼-inch rounds
- ½ cup dry white wine
- 2 tablespoons paprika
- 2 teaspoons kosher salt
- ½ tablespoon ground chili pepper
- 2 rosemary sprigs or 1 tablespoon dried rosemary
- 1 small lemon, thinly sliced
- ½ cup sliced pitted kalamata olives

DIRECTION:
1. Heat a large ovenproof skillet over high heat until hot, about 2 minutes. Add 1 tablespoon of olive oil and heat
2. Add the Branzino fillets, skin-side up, and sear for 2 minutes. Flip the fillets and cook. Set aside.
3. Swirl 2 tablespoons of olive oil around the skillet to coat evenly.
4. Add the garlic, scallions, tomatoes, and carrot, and sauté for 5 minutes

5. Add the wine, stirring until all ingredients are well combined. Carefully place the fish over the sauce.
6. Preheat the oven to 450°F (235°C).
7. Brush the fillets with the remaining 1 tablespoon of olive oil and season with paprika, salt, and chili pepper. Top each fillet with a rosemary sprig and lemon slices. Scatter the olives over fish and around the skillet.
8. Roast for about 10 minutes until the lemon slices are browned. Serve hot.

NUTRITION: Calories 724, 43g fat, 57g protein

Grilled Lemon Pesto Salmon

Preparation Time: 5 minutes

Cooking Time: 10 minutes

Serving: 2

INGREDIENTS:
- 10 ounces (283 g) salmon fillet
- 2 tablespoons prepared pesto sauce
- 1 large fresh lemon, sliced
- Cooking spray

DIRECTION:
1. Preheat the grill to medium-high heat. Spray the grill grates with cooking spray.
2. Season the salmon well. Spread the pesto sauce on top.
3. Make a bed of fresh lemon slices about the same size as the salmon fillet on the hot grill, and place the salmon on top of the lemon slices. Put any additional lemon slices on top of the salmon.
4. Grill the salmon for 10 minutes.
5. Serve hot.

Nutrition: Calories 316, 21g fat, 29g protein

Steamed Trout with Lemon Herb Crust

Preparation Time: 10 minutes

Cooking Time: 15 minutes

Serving: 2

INGREDIENTS:
- 3 tablespoons olive oil
- 3 garlic cloves, chopped
- 2 tablespoons fresh lemon juice
- 1 tablespoon chopped fresh mint
- 1 tablespoon chopped fresh parsley
- ¼ teaspoon dried ground thyme
- 1 teaspoon sea salt
- 1 pound (454 g) fresh trout (2 pieces)
- 2 cups fish stock

DIRECTION:
1. Blend olive oil, garlic, lemon juice, mint, parsley, thyme, and salt. Brush the marinade onto the fish.
2. Insert a trivet in the Instant Pot. Fill in the fish stock and place the fish on the trivet.
3. Secure the lid. Select the Steam mode and set the cooking time for 15 minutes at High Pressure.
4. Once cooking is complete, do a quick pressure release. Carefully open the lid. Serve warm.

Nutrition: Calories 477, 30g fat, 52g protein

Roasted Trout Stuffed with Veggies

Preparation Time: 10 minutes

Cooking Time: 25 minutes

Serving: 2

INGREDIENT:
- 2 (8-ounce) whole trout fillets
- 1 tablespoon extra-virgin olive oil
- ¼ teaspoon salt
- 1/8 teaspoon black pepper
- 1 small onion, thinly sliced
- ½ red bell pepper
- 1 poblano pepper
- 2 or 3 shiitake mushrooms, sliced
- 1 lemon, sliced

DIRECTION:
1. Set oven to 425ºF (220ºC). Coat baking sheet with nonstick cooking spray.
2. Rub both trout fillets, inside and out, with the olive oil. Season with salt and pepper.
3. Mix together the onion, bell pepper, poblano pepper, and mushrooms in a large bowl. Stuff half of this mix into the cavity of each fillet. Top the mixture with 2 or 3 lemon slices inside each fillet.
4. Place the fish on the prepared baking sheet side by side. Roast in the preheated oven for 25 minutes
5. Pullout from the oven and serve on a plate.

NUTRITION: Calories 453, 22g fat, 49g protein

Lemony Trout with Caramelized Shallots

Preparation Time: 10 minutes

Cooking Time: 20 minutes

Serving: 2

INGREDIENTS:
- Shallots:
- 1 teaspoon almond butter
- 2 shallots, thinly sliced
- Dash salt
- Trout:
- 1 tablespoon almond butter
- 2 (4-ounce / 113-g) trout fillets
- 3 tablespoons capers
- ¼ cup freshly squeezed lemon juice
- ¼ teaspoon salt
- Dash freshly ground black pepper
- 1 lemon, thinly sliced

DIRECTION:

1. For Shallots
2. Situate skillet over medium heat, cook the butter, shallots, and salt for 20 minutes, stirring every 5 minutes.
3. For Trout
4. Meanwhile, in another large skillet over medium heat, heat 1 teaspoon of almond butter.
5. Add the trout fillets and cook each side for 3 minutes, or until flaky. Transfer to a plate and set aside.

6. In the skillet used for the trout, stir in the capers, lemon juice, salt, and pepper, then bring to a simmer. Whisk in the remaining 1 tablespoon of almond butter. Spoon the sauce over the fish.
7. Garnish the fish with the lemon slices and caramelized shallots before serving.

NUTRITION: Calories 344, 18g fat, 21g protein

Easy Tomato Tuna Melts

Preparation Time: 5 minutes

Cooking Time: 4 minutes

Serving: 2

INGREDIENTS:
- 1 (5-oz) can chunk light tuna packed in water
- 2 tablespoons plain Greek yogurt
- 2 tablespoons finely chopped celery
- 1 tablespoon finely chopped red onion
- 2 teaspoons freshly squeezed lemon juice
- 1 large tomato, cut into ¾-inch-thick rounds
- ½ cup shredded Cheddar cheese

DIRECTION:
1. Preheat the broiler to High.
2. Stir together the tuna, yogurt, celery, red onion, lemon juice, and cayenne pepper in a medium bowl.
3. Place the tomato rounds on a baking sheet. Top each with some tuna salad and Cheddar cheese.
4. Broil for 3 to 4 minutes until the cheese is melted and bubbly. Cool for 5 minutes before serving.

NUTRITION: Calories 244, 10g fat, 30g protein

Mackerel and Green Bean Salad

Preparation Time: 10 minutes

Cooking Time: 10 minutes

Serving: 2

INGREDIENTS:
- 2 cups green beans
- 1 tablespoon avocado oil
- 2 mackerel fillets
- 4 cups mixed salad greens
- 2 hard-boiled eggs, sliced
- 1 avocado, sliced
- 2 tablespoons lemon juice
- 2 tablespoons olive oil
- 1 teaspoon Dijon mustard
- Salt and black pepper, to taste

DIRECTION:
1. Cook the green beans in pot of boiling water for about 3 minutes. Drain and set aside.
2. Melt the avocado oil in a pan over medium heat. Add the mackerel fillets and cook each side for 4 minutes.
3. Divide the greens between two salad bowls. Top with the mackerel, sliced egg, and avocado slices.
4. Scourge lemon juice, olive oil, mustard, salt, and pepper, and drizzle over the salad. Add the cooked green beans and toss to combine, then serve.

NUTRITION: Calories 737, 57g fat, 34g protein

Hazelnut Crusted Sea Bass

Preparation Time: 10 minutes

Cooking Time: 15 minutes

Serving: 2

INGREDIENTS:
- 2 tablespoons almond butter
- 2 sea bass fillets
- 1/3 cup roasted hazelnuts
- A pinch of cayenne pepper

DIRECTION
1. Ready oven to 425°F (220°C). Line a baking dish with waxed paper.
2. Brush the almond butter over the fillets.
3. Pulse the hazelnuts and cayenne in a food processor. Coat the sea bass with the hazelnut mixture, then transfer to the baking dish.
4. Bake in the preheated oven for about 15 minutes. Cool for 5 minutes before serving.

NUTRITION: Calories 468, 31g fat, 40g protein

Salmon Baked in Foil

Preparation time: 5 minutes

Cooking time: 25 minutes

Servings: 4

INGREDIENTS:

- 2 cups cherry tomatoes
- 3 tablespoons extra-virgin olive oil
- 3 tablespoons lemon juice
- 3 tablespoons almond butter
- 1 teaspoon oregano
- ½ teaspoon salt
- 4 (5-ounce / 142-g) salmon fillets

DIRECTIONS:

1. Preheat the oven to 400ºF (205ºC). Cut the tomatoes in half and put them in a bowl. Add the olive oil, lemon juice, butter, oregano, and salt to the tomatoes and gently toss to combine.
2. Cut 4 pieces of foil, about 12-by-12 inches each. Place the salmon fillets in the middle of each piece of foil.
3. Divide the tomato mixture evenly over the 4 pieces of salmon. Bring the ends of the foil together and seal to form a closed pocket.
4. Place the 4 pockets on a baking sheet. Bake in the preheated oven for 25 minutes. Remove from the oven and serve on a plate.

NUTRITION: Calories: 410 Fat: 32.0g Protein: 30.0g Carbs: 4.0g

Instant Pot Poached Salmon

Preparation time: 10 minutes

Cooking time: 3 minutes

Servings: 4

INGREDIENTS:
- 1 lemon, sliced ¼ inch thick
- 4 (6-ounce / 170-g) skinless salmon fillets, 1½ inches thick
- ½ teaspoon salt
- ¼ teaspoon pepper
- ½ cup water

DIRECTIONS:
1. Layer the lemon slices in the bottom of the Instant Pot. Season the salmon with salt and pepper, then arrange the salmon (skin - side down) on top of the lemon slices. Pour in the water.
2. Secure the lid. Select the Manual mode and set the cooking time for 3 minutes at High Pressure. Once cooking is complete, do a quick pressure release. Carefully open the lid. Serve warm.

NUTRITION: Calories: 350 Fat: 23.0g Protein: 35.0g Carbs: 0g

Balsamic-Honey Glazed Salmon

Preparation time : 5 minutes

Cooking time: 8 minutes

Servings: 4

INGREDIENTS:
- ½ cup balsamic vinegar
- 1 tablespoon honey
- 4 (8-ounce / 227-g) salmon fillets
- Sea salt and freshly ground pepper, to taste
- 1 tablespoon olive oil

DIRECTIONS:
1. Heat a skillet over medium-high heat. Combine the vinegar and honey in a small bowl. Season the salmon fillets with the sea salt and freshly ground pepper; brush with the honey-balsamic glaze.
2. Add olive oil to the skillet, and sear the salmon fillets, cooking for 3 to 4 minutes on each side until lightly browned and medium rare in the center. Let sit for 5 minutes before serving.

NUTRITION: Calories: 454 Fat: 17.3g Protein: 65.3g Carbs: 9.7g

Seared Salmon with Lemon Cream Sauce

Preparation time: 10 minutes

Cooking time: 20 minutes

Servings: 4

INGREDIENTS:

- 4 (5-ounce / 142-g) salmon fillets
- Sea salt and freshly ground black pepper, to taste
- 1 tablespoon extra-virgin olive oil
- ½ cup low-sodium vegetable broth
- Juice and zest of 1 lemon
- 1 teaspoon chopped fresh thyme
- ½ cup fat-free sour cream
- 1 teaspoon honey
- 1 tablespoon chopped fresh chives

DIRECTIONS:

1. Preheat the oven to 400ºF (205ºC). Season the salmon lightly on both sides with salt and pepper. Place a large ovenproof skillet over medium-high heat and add the olive oil.
2. Sear the salmon fillets on both sides until golden, about 3 minutes per side. Transfer the salmon to a baking dish and bake in the preheated oven until just cooked through, about 10 minutes.
3. Meanwhile, whisk together the vegetable broth, lemon juice and zest, and thyme in a small saucepan over medium-high heat until the liquid reduces by about one-quarter, about 5 minutes.

4. Whisk in the sour cream and honey. Stir in the chives and serve the sauce over the salmon.

NUTRITION: Calories: 310 Fat: 18.0g Protein: 29.0g Carbs: 6.0g

Tuna and Zucchini Patties

Preparation time: 15 minutes
Cooking time: 12 minutes
Servings: 4

INGREDIENTS:

- 3 slices whole-wheat sandwich bread, toasted
- 2 (5-ounce / 142-g) cans tuna in olive oil, drained
- 1 cup shredded zucchini
- 1 large egg, lightly beaten
- ¼ cup diced red bell pepper
- 1 tablespoon dried oregano
- 1 teaspoon lemon zest
- ¼ teaspoon freshly ground black pepper
- ¼ teaspoon kosher or sea salt
- 1 tablespoon extra-virgin olive oil
- Salad greens or 4 whole-wheat rolls, for serving (optional)

DIRECTIONS:

1. Crumble the toast into bread crumbs with your fingers (or use a knife to cut into ¼-inch cubes) until you have 1 cup of loosely packed crumbs.
2. Pour the crumbs into a large bowl. Add the tuna, zucchini, beaten egg, bell pepper, oregano, lemon zest, black pepper, and salt. Mix well with a fork.
3. With your hands, form the mixture into four (½-cup-size) patties. Place them on a plate, and press each patty flat to about ¾-inch thick.

4. In a large skillet over medium-high heat, heat the oil until it's very hot, about 2 minutes. Add the patties to the hot oil, then reduce the heat down to medium.
5. Cook the patties for 5 minutes, flip with a spatula, and cook for an additional 5 minutes. Serve the patties on salad greens or whole-wheat rolls, if desired.

NUTRITION: Calories: 757 Fat: 72.0g Protein: 5.0g Carbs: 26.0g

Fennel Poached Cod with Tomatoes

Preparation time: 15 minutes

Cooking time : 20 minutes

Servings: 4

INGREDIENTS:
- 1 tablespoon olive oil
- 1 cup thinly sliced fennel
- ½ cup thinly sliced onion
- 1 tablespoon minced garlic
- 1 (15-ounce / 425-g) can diced tomatoes
- 2 cups chicken broth
- ½ cup white wine
- Juice and zest of 1 orange
- 1 pinch red pepper flakes
- 1 bay leaf
- 1 pound (454 g) cod

DIRECTIONS:
1. Heat the olive oil in a large skillet. Add the onion and fennel and cook for 6 minutes, stirring occasionally, or until translucent. Add the garlic and cook for 1 minute more.
2. Add the tomatoes, chicken broth, wine, orange juice and zest, red pepper flakes, and bay leaf, and simmer for 5 minutes to meld the flavors.
3. Carefully add the cod in a single layer, cover, and simmer for 6 to 7 minutes. Transfer fish to a serving dish, ladle the remaining sauce over the fish, and serve.

NUTRITION: Calories: 336 Fat: 12.5g Protein: 45.1g Carbs: 11.0g

Baked Fish with Pistachio Crust

Preparation time: 15 minutes
Cooking time: 15-20 minutes

Servings: 4

INGREDIENTS:

- ½ cup extra-virgin olive oil, divided
- 1 pound (454 g) flaky white fish (such as cod, haddock, or halibut), skin removed
- ½ cup shelled finely chopped pistachios
- ½ cup ground flaxseed
- Zest and juice of 1 lemon, divided
- 1 teaspoon ground cumin
- 1 teaspoon ground allspice
- ½ teaspoon salt
- ¼ teaspoon freshly ground black pepper

DIRECTIONS:

1. Preheat the oven to 400ºF (205ºC). Line a baking sheet with parchment paper or aluminum foil and drizzle 2 tablespoons of olive oil over the sheet, spreading to evenly coat the bottom.
2. Cut the fish into 4 equal pieces and place on the prepared baking sheet.
3. In a small bowl, combine the pistachios, flaxseed, lemon zest, cumin, allspice, salt, and pepper. Drizzle in ¼ cup of olive oil and stir well.
4. Divide the nut mixture evenly on top of the fish pieces. Drizzle the lemon juice and remaining 2 tablespoons of olive oil over the fish and bake until cooked through, 15 to 20 minutes, depending on the thickness

of the fish. Cool for 5 minutes before
serving.

NUTRITION: Calories: 509 Fat: 41.0g Protein: 26.0g
Carbs: 9.0g

Dill Baked Sea Bass

Preparation time: 15 minutes

Cooking time: 10-15 minutes

Servings: 6

INGREDIENTS:

- ¼ cup olive oil
- 2 pounds (907 g) sea bass
- Sea salt and freshly ground pepper, to taste
- 1 garlic clove, minced
- ¼ cup dry white wine
- 3 teaspoons fresh dill
- 2 teaspoons fresh thyme

DIRECTIONS:

1. Preheat the oven to 425ºF (220ºC). Brush the bottom of a roasting pan with the olive oil. Place the fish in the pan and brush the fish with oil.
2. Season the fish with sea salt and freshly ground pepper. Combine the remaining ingredients and pour over the fish.
3. Bake in the preheated oven for 10 to 15 minutes, depending on the size of the fish. Serve hot.

NUTRITION: Calories: 224 Fat: 12.1g Protein: 28.1g Carbs: 0.9g

Sole Piccata with Capers

Preparation time: 15 minutes

Cooking time: 17 minutes

Servings: 4

INGREDIENTS:

- 1 teaspoon extra-virgin olive oil
- 4 (5-ounce / 142-g) sole fillets, patted dry
- 3 tablespoons almond butter
- 2 teaspoons minced garlic
- 2 tablespoons all-purpose flour
- 2 cups low-sodium chicken broth
- Juice and zest of ½ lemon
- 2 tablespoons capers

DIRECTIONS :

1. Place a large skillet over medium-high heat and add the olive oil. Sear the sole fillets until the fish flakes easily when tested with a fork, about 4 minutes on each side. Transfer the fish to a plate and set aside.
2. Return the skillet to the stove and add the butter. Sauté the garlic until translucent, about 3 minutes.
3. Whisk in the flour to make a thick paste and cook, stirring constantly, until the mixture is golden brown, about 2 minutes.
4. Whisk in the chicken broth, lemon juice and zest. Cook for about 4 minutes until the sauce is thickened. Stir in the capers and serve the sauce over the fish.

NUTRITION: Calories: 271 Fat: 13.0g Protein: 30.0g Carbs: 7.0g

Haddock with Cucumber Sauce

Preparation time: 15 minutes

Cooking time: 10 minutes

Servings: 4

INGREDIENTS:

- ¼ cup plain Greek yogurt
- ½ scallion, white and green parts, finely chopped
- ½ English cucumber, grated, liquid squeezed out
- 2 teaspoons chopped fresh mint
- 1 teaspoon honey
- Sea salt and freshly ground black pepper, to taste
- 4 (5-ounce / 142-g) haddock fillets, patted dry
- Nonstick cooking spray

DIRECTIONS:

1. In a small bowl, stir together the yogurt, cucumber, scallion, mint, honey, and a pinch of salt. Set aside. Season the fillets lightly with salt and pepper.
2. Place a large skillet over medium-high heat and spray lightly with cooking spray. Cook the haddock, turning once, until it is just cooked through, about 5 minutes per side.
3. Remove the fish from the heat and transfer to plates. Serve topped with the cucumber sauce.

NUTRITION: Calories: 164 Fat: 2.0g Protein: 27.0g Carbs: 4.0g

Crispy Herb Crusted Halibut

Preparation time: 15 minutes

Cooking time : 20 minutes

Servings: 4

INGREDIENTS:

- 4 (5-ounce / 142-g) halibut fillets, patted dry
- Extra-virgin olive oil, for brushing
- ½ cup coarsely ground unsalted pistachios
- 1 tablespoon chopped fresh parsley
- 1 teaspoon chopped fresh basil
- 1 teaspoon chopped fresh thyme
- Pinch sea salt
- Pinch freshly ground black pepper

DIRECTIONS:

1. Preheat the oven to 350°F (180°C). Line a baking sheet with parchment paper. Place the fillets on the baking sheet and brush them generously with olive oil.
2. In a small bowl, stir together the pistachios, parsley, basil, thyme, salt, and pepper. Spoon the nut mixture evenly on the fish, spreading it out so the tops of the fillets are covered.
3. Bake in the preheated oven until it flakes when pressed with a fork, about 20 minutes. Serve immediately.

NUTRITION: Calories: 262 Fat: 11.0g Protein: 32.0g Carbs: 4.0g

Pasta with Cherry Tomatoes and Anchovies

Preparation time: 15 minutes

Cooking time: 20 minutes

Servings: 5

INGREDIENTS:
- 10 ½ oz Spaghetti
- 1 1/8-pound Cherry tomatoes
- 9oz Anchovies (pre-cleaned)
- 2 tablespoons Capers
- 1 clove of garlic
- 1 Small red onion
- Parsley to taste
- Extra virgin olive oil to taste
- Table salt to taste
- Black pepper to taste
- Black olives to taste

DIRECTIONS:
1. Cut the garlic clove, obtaining thin slices.Cut the cherry tomatoes in 2. Peel the onion and slice it thinly.
2. Put a little oil with the sliced garlic and onions in a saucepan. Heat everything over medium heat for 5 minutes; stir occasionally.
3. Once everything has been well flavored, add the cherry tomatoes and a pinch of salt and pepper. Cook for 15 minutes.
4. Meanwhile, put a pot of water on the stove and as soon as it boils, add the salt and the pasta. Once the sauce is almost ready, add

the anchovies and cook for a couple of minutes. Stir gently.
5. Turn off the heat, chop the parsley and place it in the pan. When the pasta is cooked, strain it and add it directly to the sauce.Turn the heat back on again for a few seconds. Serve.

NUTRITION: Calories 446 Carbs 66.1g Protein 22.8g Fat 10g

Mussels with Tomatoes & Chili

Preparation time: 15 minutes

Cooking time: 12 minutes

Servings: 4

INGREDIENTS:
- 2 ripe tomatoes
- 2 tbsps. olive oil
- 1 tsp. tomato paste
- 1 garlic clove, chopped
- 1 shallot, chopped
- 1 chopped red or green chili
- A small glass of dry white wine
- Salt and pepper to taste
- 2 lbs./900 g. mussels, cleaned
- Basil leaves, fresh

DIRECTIONS:
1. Add tomatoes to boiling water for 3 minutes then drain.Peel the tomatoes and chop the flesh. Add oil to an iron skillet and heat to sauté shallots and garlic for 3 minutes.
2. Stir in wine along with tomatoes, chili, salt/pepper and tomato paste. Cook for 2 minutes then add mussels. Cover and let it steam for 4 minutes. Garnish with basil leaves and serve warm.

NUTRITION: Calories 483 Fat 15.2 g Carbs 20.4 g Protein 62.3 g

Lemon Garlic Shrimp

Preparation time: 15 minutes

Cooking time: 10 minutes

Servings: 6

INGREDIENTS:
- 4 tsps. extra-virgin olive oil, divided
- 2 red bell peppers, diced
- 2 lbs./900 g. fresh asparagus, sliced
- 2 tsps. lemon zest, freshly grated
- ½ tsp. salt, divided
- 5 garlic cloves, minced
- 1 lb./450 g. peeled raw shrimp, deveined
- 1 c. reduced-sodium chicken broth or water
- 1 tsp. cornstarch
- 2 tbsps. lemon juice
- 2 tbsps. fresh parsley, chopped

DIRECTIONS:
1. Add 2 teaspoon oil to a large skillet and heat for a minute. Stir in asparagus, lemon zest, bell pepper and salt. Sauté for 6 minutes.
2. Keep the sautéed veggies in a separate bowl. Add remaining oil in the same pan and add garlic.Sauté for 30 seconds then add shrimp. Cook for 1 minute.
3. Mix cornstarch with broth in a bowl and pour this mixture into the pan. Add salt and stir cook for 2 minutes. Turn off flame then add parsley and lemon juice. Serve warm with sautéed vegetables.

NUTRITION: Calories 204 Fat 4 g Carbs 23.6 g
Protein 17. 1 g

Pepper Tilapia with Spinach

Preparation time: 15 minutes

Cooking time: 27 minutes

Servings: 4

INGREDIENTS:
- 4 tilapia fillets, 8 oz./ 227 g. each
- 4 cups fresh spinach
- 1 red onion, sliced
- 3 garlic cloves, minced
- 2 tbsps. extra virgin olive oil
- 3 lemons
- 1 tbsp. ground black pepper
- 1 tbsp. ground white pepper
- 1 tbsp. crushed red pepper

DIRECTIONS:
1. Set the oven to preheat at 350°F/176.6°C. Place the fish in a shallow baking dish and juice two of the lemons.
2. Cover the fish in the lemon juice and then sprinkle the three types of pepper over the fish. Slice the remaining lemon and cover the fish. Bake in the oven for 20 minutes.
3. While the fish cooks, sauté the garlic and onion in the olive oil. Add the spinach and sauté for 7 more minutes. Top the fish with spinach and serve.

NUTRITION: Calories 323 Fat 11.4 g Carbs 10.4 g Protein 50 g

Spicy Shrimp Salad

Preparation time: 15 minutes

Cooking time: 0 minutes

Servings: 2

INGREDIENTS:
- ½ lb. salad shrimp, chopped
- 2 stalks celery, chopped
- ¼ cup red onion, diced
- 1 tsp. black pepper
- 1 tsp. red pepper
- 1 tbsp. lemon juice
- Dash of cayenne pepper
- 1 tbsp. olive oil
- 2 cucumbers, sliced

DIRECTIONS:
1. Combine the shrimp, celery, and onion in a bowl and mix together. In a separate bowl, whisk the oil and the lemon juice, then add red pepper, black pepper, and cayenne pepper.
2. Pour over the shrimp and mix. Serve with slices of thickly cut cucumber on it and enjoy.

NUTRITION: Calories: 245 Fat: 9g Carbs: 18.2g Protein: 27.3g

Lightning Source UK Ltd.
Milton Keynes UK
UKHW022056280721
387943UK00002B/275

9 781803 424941